Contents

ISBN 9780956793836

Foreword

Rewriting Life:

A New Science of Health and Longevity

So new – and so old that science has a long way to go.

What you are about to read are mostly my own observations. They are for the openminded. Rone™Therapy is not expected to be here for another 50 years. The Resonator in one form or another, has been here for over 100 years

"Life is to be enjoyed and help others to do the same." Author

Chapter 1

A Frail Beginning (1943-1990s)

I entered this world in 1943 under circumstances that could scarcely have been less promising—5 pounds and 7 ounces, a frail infant, jaundiced and with skin peeling away like the husk of an overripe fruit. My mother, weighed down by the relentless anxieties of wartime, imparted to me a tension that science would later affirm: distress endured in the womb leaves a lasting imprint upon a child.

By the age of eighteen months, asthma had claimed me as its own, my breaths emerging as laboured wheezes, my chest constricted as though encircled by unseen bands. In those early nights, my mother kept watch, her gaze fixed upon my faltering form, unaware that her own nervous unrest continued to echo within me. My father, striving to lighten her load, would reach a hand into my cot beside their bed, confirming my survival through the stillness, his touch a quiet comfort. To halt my ceaseless scratching of eczematous skin, he crafted cardboard splints, fastening my arms in a stiff yet tender appeal for relief—an act both simple and profoundly caring.

In 1948, with the establishment of the National Health Service, our family doctor advised my parents that my fragile health might benefit from a stay in a convalescent home at Ventnor, on the Isle of Wight. Thus, at five years old, I was sent to that sombre retreat, where I resided for five years among fellow asthmatics—none of us hearty enough to dash across the grounds, our days passed in subdued stillness, breaths heavy and strained. Speech proved an elusive gift; I stammered painfully, each word a barrier that silenced me, my thoughts locked within a reticent mind.

Education, too, presented its trials beyond the seasons lost to illness. At eleven, I sat the eleven-plus examination, an assessment intended to determine one's academic path, yet my performance fell into an ambiguous middle ground—neither a clear success nor an outright failure. For those of us in such a position, an oral examination followed, a prospect for which no one, it seems, had accounted for individuals like myself, burdened by a persistent stammer. I stood before three examiners, a trio of stern figures seated at a polished table, and found myself utterly incapable of articulating even my own name—each attempt a faltering gasp, my tongue ensnared by nerves. With a mixture of pity and impatience, they pronounced it for me, setting a pattern that persisted throughout the ordeal. They posed their questions, and when words eluded me, they supplied answers on my behalf, to which I could only nod in affirmation—yes—when correct. At times, they ventured incorrect responses, prompting a shake of my head—

no—an awkward dance of gesture over speech. Remarkably, despite this charade—or perhaps because of their leniency—I emerged with a pass, that ushered me into grammar school, where further challenges awaited.

Grammar school offered opportunity but was equally taxing as I forfeited three months each summer to coughing and wheezing, my allergies to the dust and pollen of the twentieth century rendering me a perennial invalid. I departed at sixteen with a solitary O-level in English Language, the sole fruit of two examinations attempted, the rest undone by pneumonia that struck just as exam week commenced, leaving me breathless and bedridden.

In 1960, I secured a position at DER, a large television rental company repairing television sets, and became their youngest outside engineer at eighteen—a role I relished for its precision and the freedom of driving from house to house, repairing sets to grateful families.

Yet, after two years, a restless spirit stirred within me, and I left, seeking something undefined beyond the routine. My adult years unfolded as a pattern of disorder—three marriages, the first two barren and fruitless, a result of my own shortcomings, as a doctor later confirmed, my sperm count too meagre to sustain life. Those unions unravelled slowly; my first wife, as insecure as I was, endured my ignorance of her needs, our evenings descending into shouting matches that tore us apart beyond mending. The second, a lovely lady, eventually wearied of my ill-tempered ways, our love fading like mist before the morning sun. At 43, and with my third wife another beautiful and lovely soul, a simple vitamin rectified nature's lapse, ——conception swiftly followed, yielding two children, now in their thirties, a belated gift. Yet I squandered that too; by 1993, my temper and reckless decisions depleted her patience, and she left, rightfully so, leaving me to face a mirror reflecting a man incapable of steadiness, my children's distant existence my only anchor against despair. Years later, I understood my anger as a futile shield against my health's failings—alas, it achieved the reverse, deepening my isolation.

Amid this chaos, I found a measure of calm in continuing as a driving instructor, a vocation I pursued on and off for thirty years. During the 1970s, I noted a clear distinction among my pupils: women learner drivers proceeded with caution, an instinct for self-preservation guiding their every manoeuvre, while most men drove with abandon, heedless of danger. Then a shift occurred—some women began to mirror the boldness of men. I attributed this to the contraceptive pill, introduced in the late 1960s, which seemed to diminish their natural wariness. In those days, it was acceptable to inquire if a pupil was using it; I ceased asking when the change became unmistakable, their driving a mirror of male audacity. Scientific studies in the 1990s later confirmed my observation, linking the contraceptive pill to heightened testosterone—a quiet vindication of my roadside insight, discerned twenty years prior as I guided ladies along the open road, a subtle triumph of an attentive mind. Yet my physical condition remained indifferent to such perceptions.

By the age of 52, in 1995, I was a veritable wreck—my lungs operated at half capacity, registering 350 on a blow medical device, my teeth fell away like leaves in autumn, and my hips groaned with arthritic protests audible with each step. Allergies persisted—eczema flared, and I wheezed at dust, pollen, the very breath of the modern era. Pneumonia had struck twice, each assault a suffocating ordeal within my chest, nights spent feverish in sweat-drenched sheets. Chest infections recurred twice yearly, as regular as the seasons—winter and summer alike ushered in by ceaseless coughing. A doctor in 1959, erring in her guidance, recommended smoking to ease my asthma; I followed her advice until 1983, when wisdom prevailed, though the harm endured—mild chronic obstructive pulmonary disease, a smoker's inheritance borne by a man who had trusted folly.

At that juncture, I teetered on an abyss—52, staring into darkness, weighing the prospect of ending it all. Solitary evenings stretched endlessly, the quiet of my home punctuated only by the clink of a bottle as I pondered a swift exit. My children, distant yet vivid in memory, held me back, their images a slender thread of light in the shadows. There was no dignity in disintegration—only a reflection of a burden upon society, my family, and myself. Doctors grew accustomed to my presence—nurses addressed me by name, a familiarity devoid of pride, my regular visits taxing their care. My kin worried, encumbered by a man who climbed stairs

with the laboured huff of an old engine. I had indulged in poor fare—pies, chips, whatever was convenient—and sat until stiffness seized me, blind to the reality that youth is a transient endowment, its accounting demanded at 40 by those who neglect it.
Allow me this observation, and heed it closely: we arrive in this world delicate, or nearly so, bearing trillions of bacteria—silent harbingers of decay—latent within us from the outset. I failed to recognise this—not at eighteen repairing televisions, not at twenty teaching drivers, not at fifty with newfound offspring, even today few are in the know.

It took decades, a wearisome journey through hardship, to grasp an essential truth: to allow oneself to falter is a selfish deed, unambiguous in its outcome. At 52, I placed a strain upon society; my children deserved a father unbroken by defeat, yet I was a man diminished. Still, one may redirect one's course—live with purpose rather than languish. At 81, I stand as proof—your days are numbered, and the age of 40 signals the hour of choice. Rise, confront your weaknesses, lest you weigh upon us all. I lingered at that brink—near ruin—and I assure you, it is a road not worth travelling.

Chapter 2

A Path Emerges (Late 1990s-2000)

By the late 1990s, I found myself in a most lamentable condition—past the age of fifty and sensing that my vigour had ebbed away, leaving me a diminished echo of the man I once was. My lungs rasped with each inhalation, my hips throbbed relentlessly, and my days were shadowed by a tiresome rhythm of coughing and unease that left me fatigued and disheartened. I must admit there were moments—long, solitary evenings—when I pondered whether it might be easier to relinquish the struggle entirely. Yet the memory of my children, though I saw them seldom following the upheavals of my personal life, held me steadfast, a gentle reminder of duties yet to be fulfilled.

It was on one such evening, however, that an unexpected encounter altered my course. I had accompanied a shy friend to a jive dance session—not to dance myself, for my ailments precluded such exertion, but to offer companionship as I watched from the sidelines, the lively steps unfolding before me. A gracious lady approached, her curiosity piqued by my stillness, and inquired why I refrained from joining in. I explained my frailties—my wheezing lungs, my aching joints—and she listened with a kindness that disarmed me. She then extended an invitation to a therapy workshop, introducing me to a concept that piqued my interest: Emotional Freedom Technique, or EFT, a practice some heralded as a potential salve for both emotional and physical woes.

EFT, she explained, entailed a curious method of tapping on designated points of the body—around the eyes, beneath the nose, along the hands—while concentrating on a specific source of distress. Though I harboured doubts, my desperation outweighed my scepticism, prompting me to acquire the EFT manual she recommended.

That evening, seated in my armchair with the soft glow of a lamp casting gentle shadows, I followed its guidance with care, tapping as instructed. To my quiet surprise, the piercing edge of my hip pain softened, and the suffocating tightness in my chest eased, if only temporarily. It was no panacea, certainly, but it offered a whisper of respite—a faint beam piercing the gloom that had settled over my existence. That modest relief kindled within me a resolve not to succumb, but to pursue a more lasting remedy.

I have always possessed an inquisitive nature, reluctant to accept things merely as presented, so I embarked upon this exploration with the diligence of a scholar. At the time, the internet was a nascent resource, limited yet promising, and I scoured its offerings for insights into EFT and other therapeutic approaches I might master. I supplemented this with library volumes on ancient healing traditions—from China and Egypt, centuries old—describing a vital energy flowing through us, an essence elusive to precise quantification yet resonant with intuitive truth. Contemporary medicine provided scant endorsement of such notions, but I remained undaunted by its reticence; I placed my trust in the possibility that understanding might lie beyond the bounds of conventional practice. I began helping others—friends, acquaintances, even my driving pupils—welcoming them into my home to sit over tea, tapping away their troubles: financial worries, lingering family grievances. The outcomes varied—sometimes a weight lifted, sometimes it persisted—but each small victory encouraged me to press forward. Yet I pondered: it worked, but why not consistently?

For two years, I laboured with unwavering dedication, refining the technique as I had once repaired television sets in my youth at DER, noting observations in the stillness of night until, by 2000, and using information from the varied therapies, I had perfected a method of my own—Removal of Negative Emotions, or RONE, as I termed it, a simple name for a remarkable solution. Born of patience and persistence, I designed it to dispel troubling emotions with certainty and speed. I would sit with an individual— a neighbour, perhaps, or a friend—reciting to me their burden: anger, fear, sorrow, whatever pressed upon their spirit. I sought no lengthy recounting of their hardships, only the emotion itself. I offered a clear set of instructions, spoken once, guiding them to dwell upon their distress. Then, with a brief phrase—a mantra, the emotion melted away, as though a heavy load had been gently set aside.

This process, completed in a single session of a few hours, eradicated all traces of their emotional strife. During the session I teach them to understand the workings so they may help themselves thereafter—a mere half-minute should another negative feeling arise—and since 2000, I have assisted over a thousand individuals, with all but a few finding solace, a 98% success rate that is unparalleled to this day. I called it "The most advanced talk therapy in the world." I am still waiting for someone to challenge it.

My initial trial was personal—my hips, a source of enduring torment. The left had been replaced in the late 1990s with the Birmingham hip resurfacing, akin to that later used by a renowned sportsman, skilfully managed by a masterful surgeon despite an X-ray revealing a hole in the hip the size of a five-pence piece, raising doubts about its durability. The right hip, slated for replacement a year hence, was equally wretched, bone grinding on bone, its pain at times unbearable. EFT dulled it initially, but with RONE—then newly named—I banished the pain entirely, focusing on the negative emotion causing the pain, reciting the mantra, and for twelve years I lived free of discomfort until a knee misalignment, caused by that untreated hip, necessitated its eventual replacement.

At a Mind Body Spirit show where I delivered a talk, a gentleman approached me afterward, his expression earnest, asking if I could relieve his pain. Both his hips had been surgically restored in youth, yet the left continued to afflict him, a dull agony persisting for the last fifteen years. At his session, he addressed his grievances—anger at the surgeons, anxiety over his work—yet the pain endured. We persisted, clearing past quarrels and minor fears, until he mentioned, almost casually, a slight annoyance: a neighbour's sharp remark from years ago. We concentrated there, applied the method, and to our shared astonishment, the pain vanished. He rose, tested his leg, and we exchanged a quiet chuckle—a trivial grievance had wielded such influence. He has utilised it since, a swift correction whenever negativity stirs the ache anew.

Another instance involved a lady in her thirties. She could hardly eat without her chest tightening alarmingly, as though her heart yearned to break free, reduced to subsisting on cabbage soup. Doctors detected no physical origin, but she linked it to a distressing lunch—a dispute with children as she consumed a mushroom, persuading her the food was to blame. We tackled her burdens—lost loves, that fraught meal, her dread of mushrooms—yet the sensation lingered. Probing gently, removing a deal of emotions, testing her taste after each one, she recalled a youthful romance that had ended in heartbreak. We dispelled that sorrow, and again she sampled a tiny piece of chocolate—no distress ensued. She ventured toast with butter—perfectly well, and so she remains. Over a thousand have followed—men riled by temper and anxiety, women worn by worry and care, elderly folk stooped by regret—all restored, a testament to RONE's simplicity and efficiency.

In those shadowed days of the late 1990s, I pondered an affliction from my youth, my stammer, a halting barrier that silenced me since childhood. It seemed a mirror of insecurity, for I observed in others that when this burden lifted through RONE Therapy, their speech flowed freely once more. My own voice, once faltering through nine words in ten, found respite when I began work repairing television sets at DER. There, I learned to sidestep troublesome words, easing my stammer by ninety parts in a hundred, a practical shield against my inner doubt. Yet it was RONE, devised by 2000, that brought complete liberation. I remove the insecurity from those with a stammer, together with their stumbling words. The process reveals a truth: the mind's unrest shapes even our words, and in its calm, lies freedom.

RONE did not wholly mend my physical frame—my lungs still rasped; my chest seized at times—but it lifted me from a shadowed abyss. Before RONE, I was a drain—doctors tired of my presence, family strained by my weakness. I had sat alone, bitter at my fate, fearful of its end, a weight upon those near me. RONE dissolved that darkness—anger and dread faded—granting a clarity absent for decades. It addressed the mind, not the body, yet the mind constitutes half the battle, and I had been losing it grievously. It took nearly fifty years to apprehend this truth: a sound life commences within. By 2000, I ceased encumbering others—instead, I uplifted them, over a thousand restored to brighter days. You may do likewise—cast off your mind's burdens, stand tall, spare others your strain. At 81, I stand as proof—born frail, I found a path, and it is yours should you choose to follow.

Chapter 3

A New Device (2018 Onwards)

By 2018, I had attained the age of 74, a milestone at which many might acquiesce to the gradual waning of their years, yet I found myself resolute in a new dimension, my mental clarity for nearly two decades, dispelling the shadows of anger and fear that once darkened my existence. Nevertheless, my physical condition persisted as an unrelenting adversary. Although I had rid myself of my asthma and allergies with RONE, I was still plagued with chest infections and bronchitis every year relying on antibiotics. It was not in my character to sit passively, mourning what could not be reversed; thus, when a colleague suggested a visit to a lady from Ukraine who offered a bio-resonance device, I approached the prospect with cautious curiosity. She claimed it could remedy bodily ailments through vibrations—a concept both novel and faintly improbable, yet intriguing enough to warrant investigation.

I arranged to meet her at her home one crisp morning, where she welcomed me with a warm smile and demonstrated the device. Seated in her dining room, I underwent a session, attaching the apparatus to my hands as she directed, its gentle hum and flickering lights the only signs of activity. After an hour, I rose, expecting some alleviation, yet my cough remained steadfast, my chest as oppressed as ever. Disappointed but not dissuaded, I nonetheless purchased one, compelled by a flicker of hope. At home, I followed the sparse instructions—holding it for an hour daily—yet the results mirrored my initial trial: no discernible change.

Undeterred, I telephoned the supplier, seeking to understand the principle behind its vibrations. Her reply was vague—she could not elucidate it fully—but she recommended I explore the works of Dr.

Hulda Clark, a name then unknown to me, sparking a new avenue of inquiry. Intrigued, I watched a video online featuring Clark and subsequently purchased her first book, "The Cure For All Diseases". That evening, I settled with a cup of tea, prepared to examine her propositions with an open yet discerning mind. Clark's argument was striking—she asserted that a host of afflictions, from coughs to more severe conditions, originated from microscopic parasites and bacteria dwelling within us, susceptible to eradication through one precise vibrational frequency. It struck me as a remarkable assertion, yet not entirely implausible; my experience with RONE had taught me that unconventional approaches might hold value where traditional methods faltered.

Emboldened, I sought one of Clark's devices and discovered a gentleman who crafted what she termed a zapper in his garden shed, originally for his daughter and her friends. I ordered one online, and it arrived—a compact box to be powered by a 9-volt battery, equipped with two copper handles. Following Clark's guidance, I seated myself in my armchair and grasped the handles—ten minutes on, a twenty-minute rest, repeated three times daily, a cycle I maintained for several days. Each day, a chest infection that had gripped me for weeks—what some called the "thirty-day cough"—began to subside. I coughed vigorously, expelling a substantial amount of phlegm, and within days it had vanished, a swiftness unprecedented in my long history of such maladies. Astonished, I telephoned the craftsman, my gratitude tempered by a growing determination. "Would you produce more?" I asked, outlining my desire to share this discovery. He hesitated— "I make them only for my girl"—but after some gentle persuasion, he consented to fashion ten within a couple of weeks.

In the spring of 2018, before the pandemic, I brought them to a lecture I delivered at a local hall, attended by curious individuals eager for further understanding. I held up an aluminium case containing the device. "In this case I have a device that destroys harmful bacteria, viruses and parasites, how much will you give for it?" I described the zapper's impact on my chest—its simplicity and potential "a thousand pounds said one" and by the session's close, all ten had found new owners, nowhere near thousand but at a reasonable price for such promise. I was selling it for what it was, not what it did. Some remarked that "zapper" sounded abrupt, prompting me to reflect over supper; I settled upon "Resonator"—a name both refined and suggestive of its function.

Determined to enhance it, I engaged a small factory to produce the device with precision—operating at 30 kilohertz, a frequency of 30 vibrations per second, powered by a 9-volt battery, its reliability ensured by technical supervision. I began offering them—ninety-seven pounds with postage through a website I established, www.resonator.uk, seventy pounds at the Mind Body Spirit fairs I frequented, and one free for every two sold, a gesture to aid those in need but short of means. The Resonator kills harmful bacteria and parasites and destroys viruses with its minute vibrations, targeting even the smallest pathogens. No further need for antibiotics or vaccines—I, and everyone I know who uses one, stand as living testimony to that claim.

Over six years, more than 200 have been distributed, with only two returned—one by an elderly lady disconcerted by its sensation, another by a young woman who deemed it ineffective. For me, the benefits transcended that initial relief—my sense of smell, dulled for decades, returned with remarkable clarity, the smell of cooking once again a joy; nocturnal spasms in my neck, which had plagued my rest, ceased entirely after consistent use. Losing one's sense of smell, is now known as an early herald of brain afflictions—dementia, Parkinson's, and more. Studies point to bacteria as the culprits, their sole purpose to consume, gnawing at the mind's fabric when pH falters. Dementia's bacterial scent and loss of smell begins, as mine did, reversed by the Resonator.

I must point out that bacteria are very small. 50 billion can be found in a probiotic capsule—twenty and you have 1 trillion. A trillion seconds is 31,000 years, and viruses—10 to 100 times smaller. their tiny size is beyond most people's comprehension.

In 2019 at the beginning of the pandemic, I advertised the Resonator on Facebook as an alternative to vaccines for those who could or would not take a vaccine. The abuse I suffered in those two weeks was astounding, they would not understand that the Resonator destroyed the virus. One was purchased by an agent of the MHRA who complained to the ASA. They in turn banned me from advertising as they had two complaints, an individual and the MHRA. I had already stopped advertising, but the ASA published my ban which is still out there, stating that I was irresponsible and stopping people from using the vaccines. Since then, it has only been distributed at MBS fairs and by word of mouth.

I adopted a new routine with the Resonator—fifteen minutes every other day initially, now fifteen to thirty minutes daily—a practice that has sustained me without a single cold, let alone a chest infection. A cherished friend, aged 90, encountered a dire predicament—an ill-suited hospital pill for his prostate, unsuitable for an elderly man with low blood pressure, triggered a cardiac collapse. Within two weeks, he diminished from ten stone to seven, a frail figure confined to a bed. His doctors abandoned hope; his daughter telephoned me in anguish, certain he would not return home. I had given him a Resonator many years ago, which he used fifteen minutes daily at the start of his pain, prior to his hospital ordeal.

A week later, his voice reached me over the phone—normal and resolute, a survivor, a walking skeleton, now reliant on a walking frame. We concluded the device had reduced the bacterial burden so much, there were too few left to continue their progressive act of consuming the body as the cellular oxygen depleted. Today, despite irreversible heart damage, he has recovered—a testament to the Resonator's potency.

Other testimonies—a lady in her fifties attended a fair with a stubborn cough, reporting it vanquished after three days of fifteen-minute sessions; a man with a leg wound slow to heal found it swiftly restored within a week. A family texted me— "Myself at 72, my husband at 77, and our asthmatic daughter contracted a bout of COVID-19. I found the Resonator, and we shared it, each using it for ten minutes, rotating it between us for four and a half hours. We emerged clear in two days, save my daughter's lingering cough for a fortnight." Many such accounts have reached me—coughs relieved, pains eased, senses rejuvenated—each a quiet confirmation of this device's value. My own chest infections, a biannual affliction since 1948, have not recurred in six years, a liberation I scarcely imagined possible.

These successes are not solely mine—they belong to those who seized the chance, and they illuminate a broader principle: one need not surrender to the frailties time imposes. Before RONE, I encumbered society—doctors bore my frequent visits, my family shouldered my decline; with the Resonator, I have supported over 200, complementing the thousand uplifted by RONE. It is a matter of straightforward reason—to reject dependency and offer aid to others. At 81, I stand as proof—born frail, I have journeyed from infirmity to purpose across nearly seven decades. This Resonator, a modest spark, extends the same to you—sustain your health, diminish the reaper's unseen helpers, and live with dignity. It is yours to embrace, should you choose to do so.

Chapter 4

Insights That Endure

Why Age 40 Marks the Divide

By the time the Resonator became a fixture in my life—2018, when I was 74—I found myself pondering more deeply the reasons behind its efficiency, and indeed, why my health had faltered so grievously in earlier years. RONE Therapy, perfected by 2000, had sustained my mental clarity for nearly two decades, banishing the anger and fear that once overshadowed my existence, removing my allergies and asthma. The Resonator, I found eighteen years later, quelled my chest infections and restored faculties dulled by time—my sense of smell, my restful nights—offering a physical reprieve where RONE had fortified my mind.

Yet questions lingered: why had my body succumbed so readily before, and why did these tools succeed where conventional remedies faltered? Clark's assertions, which I had first encountered through her video and writings, posited those countless ailments—from persistent coughs to dire conditions—arose from microscopic parasites and bacteria harboured within us, destroyed by vibrational frequencies. Jerry Tennant in his "Healing is Voltage" book, suggested we are born with trillions of bacteria, inherent companions that remain dormant until awakened by a shift in our body's balance pH. pH, a measure of acidity or alkalinity on a scale from 1 to 14, with 7 as neutral. A healthy individual, maintains a pH around 7.3, slightly alkaline; when this balance dips, oxygen diminishes, and these bacteria stir, consuming us from within—lungs, joints, organs, wherever they find a malfunction to feed. Both theories struck me as compelling, resonating with my own history: chest infections twice yearly since 1948, hips grinding by 52, a body beleaguered until RONE and the Resonator intervened.

Reflecting over my tea, I recalled the Resonator's swift dispersal of my "thirty-day cough" in 2018—a liberation antibiotics had never achieved—and my friend at 90, whose dwindling frame refused to die, rallied after a hospital misstep, his prior daily fifteen-minute sessions leaving too few bacteria to claim him. A lady at a fair, her cough vanquished in three days; another with pains eased after weeks—over 200 such instances affirmed Clark's claim of vibrational purging. Yet Tennant's pH notion lingered, prompting me to consider a pattern I had observed across decades, particularly at the Mind Body Spirit fairs where I shared these tools. Three ladies, all under 40, approached me one spring day, each bearing a diagnosis of breast cancer—nothing else amiss, no coughs, no aches, just that singular affliction. Tennant wrote that cancer emerges when pH falls below 5.5, cells starved of oxygen turning rogue, yet these women showed no signs of bacterial awakening—no joint pains, no infections. It set me wondering: why the discrepancy?

I turned my thoughts to those I had aided with RONE—over a thousand since 2000, many under 40 grappling with emotional distress—tight chests from worry, heads clouded by sorrow—yet their bodies remained robust, free of the ailments that plagued me past 50. Older individuals at the fairs—beyond 40, often weary and unwell—found swift relief with the Resonator, their coughs and pains receding, while younger attendees sometimes reported no effect, their vigour intact. One evening, I pieced it together: 40 marks a divide, a threshold in our vitality. Before 40, our bodies hold firm—bacteria dormant—even amidst emotional tempests where the pH could be way below normal. After 40, neglect tips the balance, pH has faltered, and those silent agents awaken. An adage came to mind—"The body looks after you until you are 40, then you must look after your body"—

echoed by history: a century ago, before antibiotics. 40 was a common lifespan, a natural pivot from resilience to decline.

This notion crystallised as I sipped my tea, recalling my own descent at 52—lungs half-functional, hips arthritic, chest infections relentless—contrasted with my vigour at 40, teaching drivers despite asthma's grip. Stress, drives pH downward, releasing cortisol—a hormone thickening blood against injury, yet rendering it acidic, souring cells and rousing bacteria.

My years of anger—shouting matches with my first wife, temper fraying my third marriage—had surely fuelled that sourness, a realisation dawning decades too late. RONE purged that stress, lifting my mind's burden and removing the associated pains: the Resonator quelled the bacterial aftermath, yet I wondered: why 40?

Sportsmen lose their edge, some retire near that age—late thirties, early forties—their peak fading as unseen forces stir. At a fair, a lady in her fifties spoke of her husband's cough, unrelenting until the Resonator intervened, while her daughter, under 40, shrugged off ailments with ease—pH held firm in youth, faltered in age if untended. Children are better equipped with a higher pH than the normal 7.3, often more than 8.

Clark's parasites intrigued me further—endometriosis, she claimed, stemmed from misplaced parasites, a theory borne out by a woman in her forties at a fair, her pains of years vanishing after a few days with the Resonator, hinting at a child now possible. Yet those under 40 cancer cases—pH low, bacteria asleep—suggested a split: Youth withstands emotional strain, age invites bacterial revolt if you fail to look after your body.

As I pondered the delicate balance of pH, a subtle yet striking observation emerged, one rooted in the simplest of human exchanges. A kiss, that brief mingling of fluids, reveals much to a woman about the man she meets. Within a fleeting moment, her senses discern a taste, sweet or bitter, a verdict delivered in milliseconds. Should he be a stranger and the taste prove bitter, she recoils, her instinct urging no further encounter. If sweet, she proceeds with ease, a silent affirmation of his wellness.

Yet in a bond long formed, a kiss once sweet turning bitter signals a shift, a sign that acidity has crept into his frame. Something has unsettled him, perhaps a quiet upset or a deeper trauma, altering his inner harmony. To probe this change, a simple test suffices, a saliva check with pH strips, those modest tools revealing whether his balance dips below the healthy mark of 7.3. Such bitterness, I found, often heralds the stirring of bacteria, a clue to unrest that my own methods later quelled. This humble kiss, a whisper of nature's wisdom, offers a window into vitality, a lesson in how closely our wellness intertwines with the unseen currents within us.

Another observation is alcohol. It appears the more negative emotions one has, the more alcohol one can consume before effects. After a Rone session, one can take very little before it affects.

Over tea with a friend one afternoon, I mused aloud—my chest infections ceased at 74 with the Resonator, my friend at 90 endured, yet young folk bore no such loads until later. My hypothesis — that low pH before 40, allows most bodies to carry on. After 40 — it's like a switch. If the pH is low, then the oxygen would be low, and the dormant bacteria awake, the lower the pH, the more bacteria awake. The Resonator silenced bacteria—RONE removes the negative emotions that cause the acidity, together they defied the decline. If the bacteria lie dormant, doing no harm for forty years, why does it awaken after forty? My hypothesis is that our lives should end just after 40, it did a hundred years ago. Antibiotics have extended that time, but eventually we succumb to the ravages of the bacteria.

Sports people, especially those at top of their game, feel the stress of being, doubting themselves when beaten into second. The stresses mean nothing to the fit under 40s, but past, the edge falls away because the reapers little helpers have awakened. More stress, more wake, slowly you start to lose the accuracy you had, all caused by doubt. You retire before you are retired.

These insights, distilled over years, bore a practical truth. Big firms—pharmaceutical giants—scorn such simplicity; the Resonator threatens their pill-driven profits, just as RONE's guarantee, no mend, no fee, defies costly therapies. Health authorities halted my notices—demanding marks of approval, unobtainable trials at a million a trial, proven harmless. Over 200 Resonators and a thousand RONE sessions speak louder than their silence. Only two returned the device—one unsettled, one unconvinced—while the rest endure, a quiet chorus of efficiency. 40 is your moment—before, your mind may falter, yet your frame holds; after, bacteria will rise if you slacken. I saw it in those young cancer patients—pH fell, yet no bugs stirred—versus my ruin past 40, halted only by intervention.

At 81, I reflect on this divide—my chest once a battleground, now calm; my mind, once shadowed, now clear. It took nearly seven decades to discern: stress sours you, pH wakes the reaper's helpers, and 40 is the hinge. RONE lifts the spirit, Resonator quells the foe—both sustain dignity where I once burdened society. Doctors weary of me faded from my life; my kin no longer bear my weight. You need not falter as I did—heed your forty, tend your balance, spare others your load. I stand as evidence—born frail, I faltered, yet rose. These tools, these truths, are yours—embrace them, help your fellows, and keep the reaper at bay a while longer.

Chapter 5

Stories That Affirm

By the time RONE Therapy and the Resonator had become integral to my existence—the former since 2000, the latter from 2018—I had encountered a host of individuals whose lives bore the marks of struggle, much like my own, yet who found renewal through these tools. Over a thousand had sought RONE's clarity, their minds unburdened in a single session, while more than 200 had embraced the Resonator, with one gratis for every two sold—a gesture to extend aid where means were scant. Only two returned the device—one unsettled by its sensation, another unconvinced—leaving a chorus of over 200 whose experiences, alongside my own, testified to its worth. These were not mere transactions; they were encounters, often, where I listened, offered what I had learned, and witnessed transformations that affirmed the path I had forged. Here, I recount a few such stories—

not as boasts, but as evidence that one need not languish, and that dignity can replace dependency.

One spring afternoon, a gentleman approached me following a talk at a Mind Body Spirit fair, his face etched with weariness. He introduced himself—let us call him Mr. Carter, for discretion's sake—in his late forties, a man whose youth had been marred by surgical replacements of both hips, a necessity that left his left side aching fifteen years on. Physicians had exhausted their explanations, deeming it sound, yet the dull torment persisted, robbing him of rest.

During his session I inquired into his troubles—not the full tale, but the emotions beneath: anger at the surgeons who had failed him, anxiety over his livelihood strained by pain. With RONE, we addressed these—focusing on each, reciting the mantra—yet the ache lingered. We pressed on, clearing old quarrels and minor fears, until he mentioned, almost offhandedly, a neighbour's curt remark from years past, a trivial slight that had festered. We turned our attention there, applied the method, and to our mutual astonishment, the pain lifted entirely. He rose, tested his leg, and we shared a quiet laugh—a fleeting grievance had wielded such enduring power. He has relied on it since, a swift remedy when negativity stirs the ache anew.

Another encounter came via a phone call when a lady in her thirties—let us name her Miss Evans—arrived at my home, her expression taut with worry, settling on my sofa with a warm glass of water. She could scarcely eat without her chest tightening alarmingly, as though her heart sought to break free, confining her to a diet of cabbage soup. Doctors found no physical cause, but she traced it to a distressing lunch—a squabble with children as she ate a mushroom, convincing her the food was the culprit. We explored her burdens—removed them one by one, lost loves, that unhappy meal, her dread of mushrooms—yet the sensation persisted. Gently probing further, she recalled a youthful romance that had ended in heartbreak, a wound still tender beneath her composure. We focused there, recited the mantra, and the sorrow dissolved. She ventured a piece of chocolate—no distress followed. She tried toast with butter—perfectly well, and so she has remained. Over the following weeks, she regained her confidence in nourishment, a quiet triumph of mind over affliction, one of over a thousand I have guided since 2000, all restored by this simple clarity.

Across my years, I have met many men and women bearing the scars of indignities—cruel blows that left them shadowed by trauma for decades. Their disgust, anger, and silent wounds, etched deep, found release in a single session of RONE Therapy., I guided them to name their burdens—no lengthy tales required, merely the emotion itself—

anger, shame, despair. dissolved, astonishment lighting their faces as peace took root. Even I, at times, marvel at RONE's reach. Ex-soldiers, hardened by sights no man should endure—war's indelible mark of terror and loss—came to me, their anguish lifted in hours, the spectre of sleepless nights banished.

All manner of dark feelings—grief, dread, hopelessness—yielded to this method. Among them were those long bowed by depression, tethered to medications for years, who awoke after their RONE session to a new dawn, casting aside their pills. Withdrawal proved gentle, a whisper rather than a storm, for the chief culprits—negative emotions—had been swept away. These individuals, once resigned to shadow, stood anew, their vitality a quiet testament to RONE's power, a gift I share not as pride, but as proof that renewal lies within reach for all who seek it.

The Resonator, too, wove its own tales. One autumn day, the daughter of a cherished friend—aged 90—telephoned me in distress, her voice trembling with fear that he would not return home. A hospital pill for his prostate, ill-suited for an elderly man with low blood pressure, had precipitated a cardiac collapse, reducing him from ten stone to seven in a mere fortnight, a fragile figure confined to a bed. His doctors had relinquished hope, yet I had given him a Resonator months prior to this ordeal, which he used fifteen minutes daily. A week later, his voice reached me over the line—normal and resolute, a survivor now reliant on a walking frame. We surmised the device had diminished the bacterial load sufficiently to spare him; he persisted with it, and today, despite irreversible heart damage, he has recovered, a living testament to its efficiency. I recall our tea together months later, his gratitude palpable as he described his return to pottering about—a life reclaimed where medicine had faltered.

Another lady, in her fifties—let us call her Mrs. Jones—approached me at a fair, her persistent cough a shadow over her days. She acquired a Resonator, reporting three days later that three fifteen-minute sessions daily had vanquished it entirely, a relief she described with quiet joy over the telephone. A man—Mr. Harris, for our purposes—suffered a leg wound slow to heal, yet found it swiftly mended within a week of daily use, marvelling at its speed in a shower of thanks. Then came a family's account, relayed via text: "Myself at 72, my husband at 77, our asthmatic daughter contracted a bout of COVID-19. I found the Resonator, and we shared it—each using it for ten minutes, passing it to the next, continuing for just over four and a half hours. We emerged clear in two days, save my daughter's lingering cough for a fortnight.

One autumn day, I delivered a lecture on RONE Therapy to a gathering of ex-forces personnel, a group seasoned by life's rigors, their faces etched with tales of endurance. Afterward, an elderly gentleman approached me, his gait cautious, his eyes searching—let us call him Mr. Thompson for discretion's sake. He inquired whether I could relieve a back pain that had tormented him for eight years, born of a fall from a small stepladder while replacing a lightbulb. He had landed squarely, yet the impact damaged his spine, an injury that defied the efforts of the finest doctors from Harley Street down, right across the country, none able to grant him respite despite his persistent quest.

To ease his burden, I arranged to visit him at his home, where we sat in his quiet sitting room. We embarked upon the task of uncovering his relief. We began with tracing his past sorrows—anger, fear, regrets. Each emotion focused upon was released with the RONE. Then we addressed the pain itself, yet it lingered stubbornly, an unyielding companion. "There must be something else you have not recalled," I suggested gently, sensing a deeper root. He paused, then shared a story I had encountered before—two sons, paths divergent. The elder excelled—university, a career in London's financial heart, success in his father's eyes; the younger sought his own way, faltering with intermittent work, struggling to thrive. He had sought his father's aid, only to be rebuffed for defying paternal expectations. "How do you feel about that?" I asked. "Guilty," he murmured, "perhaps I should have done more." We turned to that guilt, clearing it alongside other sentiments tied to his second son—regret, disappointment—removing them all, I asked him to stand and assess his pain. He rose and stood silently; tears started tracing his weathered cheeks. "The pain has gone," he said, voice trembling, "for the first time in eight years, I have no pain."

I have witnessed this pattern often—and concluded, that nearly all pain lingering beyond a year from accidents or mishaps reveals itself as emotional. The emotion manifesting itself mostly in the weakest part of the body, a burden of the mind masquerading as bodily affliction. Many have found pain relief through RONE, yet two cases stand apart: one lady clung to her pain for secondary gain, its presence a shield; another, a man summoned by his daughter, wielded his discomfort as a pretext to avoid work. I saw him without prior discussion, a rarity—for now I insist on speaking with each individual first, ensuring their earnest desire for recovery. Mr. Thompson's tears affirmed a truth: emotional wounds, left untended, exact a physical toll, yet they too can be lifted, restoring dignity where once there was despair. Simply remove the negative emotion.

These accounts—Mr. Carter's laugh, Miss Evans' toast, my friend's resolute voice, Mr. Thompson's tearful relief—form a quiet chorus with over 200 who embraced the

Resonator and over a thousand restored by RONE, my own journey woven among them. My chest infections, a biannual scourge since 1948, ceased six years ago with the Resonator's daily use—fifteen to thirty minutes now sustaining me without a cold, my sense of smell sharp once more, nocturnal spasms a memory. Before RONE, I was a burden—doctors weary of my presence, my family strained by my frailty; before the Resonator, my body faltered despite a cleared mind. These tools together shifted my course—each story a thread in a tapestry of renewal, shared with me over on my sofa or MSB fairs chats, affirming a truth I grasped after decades: one need not succumb to infirmity.

These accounts underscore a principle I hold dear: we need not impose our frailties upon society. At 52, I drained resources—doctors knew me by name, my kin bore my weight; at 81, I stand unencumbered, aiding others rather than encumbering them. It took nearly seven decades—born frail, faltering at midlife—to discern this path. RONE lifts the spirit's load, the Resonator quells the body's foes—together, they offer dignity where I once knew despair. You need not follow my earlier course—burdening those around you with neglect—but may choose renewal instead. At fairs, I've seen it—young old people restored by RONE, and the Resonator—each a step from dependency to contribution. These stories, over a thousand strong, are evidence—mine among them—that you too can rise, spare others your strain, and extend a hand. It is yours to claim, should you wish it so.

Chapter 6
The Complete Design

By 2018, with the Resonator running alongside RONE Therapy—tools I had honed since 2000 and 2018 respectively—I found myself at 74, piecing together a broader pattern that had sustained me beyond the frailties of my youth. Born in 1943, a frail infant at 5 pounds and 7 ounces, I had weathered asthma, chest infections, and a body that faltered grievously by 52—lungs half-gone, hips arthritic, a burden to doctors and kin alike. Yet at 81, I stood renewed, my chest clear for six years, my mind shadowed, a man no longer draining society but aiding it—over a thousand lifted by RONE, over 200 by the Resonator. One evening, sat in my reclining armchair, I reflected on this transformation—not a single stroke of fortune financially, but a treasure trove by design, a complete circle of practices that had turned decline into vigour. It was not merely the tools, but a way of living—mind, body, and habits aligned—that offered this reprieve, a path I share here, not as a boast, but as an invitation to others.

RONE Therapy, born of my late 1990s despair, was the cornerstone—over a thousand souls, from Mr. Carter with his aching hip to Mr. Thompson with his tearful relief, found clarity in a single session, their burdens of anger, fear, and guilt dissolved. My own mind, once a mire of resentment, anger, fear, worry—shouting matches with my first wife, temper fraying my third—cleared at 57, lifting a weight that had soured me for decades. It took two years well spent, to banish those shadows, a practice I've helped others to sustain in half a minute should distress resurface. Yet my body lingered in ruin—lungs rasping, chest seizing—until the Resonator arrived in 2018, a marvel from a shed craftsman's ingenuity, refined to run at 30 kilohertz. Fifteen to thirty minutes daily silenced my biannual infections, restored my sense of smell, and quelled nocturnal spasms—a physical renewal where RONE had fortified my spirit, my emotional and physical pain.

These tools alone, however, were but pieces of a greater whole. At 52, I had gorged on pies and chips, sat until stiffness claimed me, my pH—my body's balance—souring, rousing bacteria to feast. By 2018, I understood: food matters. I shed two stone in three weeks—not a boast, but a method I detailed in "How I Lost 2 Stone in 3 Weeks", an Amazon book born of necessity. No more rubbish—fresh vegetables, meats, fruits, and coconut oil replaced the seed oils and haste of my youth. One afternoon, preparing a meal of steamed broccoli, carrots, sweet potatoes, and green beans, I marvelled at the simplicity—nourishment that sustained rather than sapped. Exercise followed naturally—not grand feats a couple of hundred jumps on my rebounder and five minutes on my stepper countering the idleness that had once shackled me. My hips, bone on bone for twelve years with RONE's relief, moved easier with each step, a rhythm that fortified my frame where once it crumbled.

Supplements, too, played their part—a lesson from my fifties, when vitamin E sparked life where none had been, granting me two children now in their thirties. At 74, I added others—vitamin C, D3 K2, calcium with zinc and magnesium and phytoplankton that modern food alone will miss, a quiet nod to nature's gaps. Over tea with a friend one day, he remarked on my vigour— "You've outpaced us all"—and I smiled, knowing these small tablets, alongside diet and movement, had plugged holes time might otherwise widen.

In reflecting upon the elements that sustain vitality, I turned to a curious insight about blood groups, long substantiated by Dr. Peter D'Adamo in his book, "Eat Right 4

Your Type", which I encountered in 2000. He demonstrated that each blood group, A, B, AB, and O, thrives on certain foods and must avoid others, a principle I found compelling. He suggested too that these groups might shape one's outlook on life, prompting me to ask every client their blood type before their RONE Therapy sessions. Soon, I perceived a pattern confirming his view. Blood groups not only influence mentality but also physical form, a revelation that struck me as both simple and profound. Type A individuals often appeared steadfast, their resolve unyielding until emotions released, while Type O clients burned with a fiercer spirit, their tempers cooling under RONE's guidance.

If foods affect blood groups differently, I mused, might not drugs follow a similar course? For those that must endure a tedious procession of medications for a single ailment, trial after trial, until one suits them, a wasteful ordeal. A pill taken once, then discarded, repeats needlessly, costing the National Health Service millions. A remedy lies within reach. Let doctors first determine each patient's blood group, then maintain a simple database listing the four types alongside effective drugs. For a Type O patient, the physician selects a known suitable remedy, recording it in the O column. An unsuitable drug joins an adjacent list, and so forth across A, B, and AB. Over time, a clear guide emerges, revealing which drugs align with each group. Exceptions will arise, duly noted, yet even these may share common traits. Drug firms may bristle at such clarity, but the savings in resources and relief to patients would be immense, a practical step toward wellness rooted in nature's own design.

This design—RONE for the mind, Resonator for bacteria, diet, exercise, supplements, blood type wisdom—unfolded over decades, each piece a response to my frailties. At 52, I was a wreck—doctors knew me, my family fretted—yet at 81, I burden no one. My friend at 90, spared by the Resonator; Miss Evans, eating freely; Mr. Thompson, tearfully pain-free—over 200 and a thousand, respectively, echo my renewal. One evening, testing myself with an IHeart device that tells you the biological age of your arteries, I found my arteries at 54, my rest heart rate steady at 58 beats a minute—proof at 81 of a body decades younger, a circle completed. Big firms scorn it—no profit in such simplicity; health authorities halted my notices, yet the chorus of lives restored drowns their silence.

The age 40 marks the hinge, as I learned—before, youth shields you, pH firm, bacteria dormant; after, neglect sours you, cortisol wakes them. My 52 was ruin—stress, idleness, poor fare—yet this design reversed it. RONE lifts stress, Resonator quells bacteria, diet and exercise balance pH, supplements and blood types refine it—a harmony that spares society my load. I've seen it—young and old folk cleared by RONE, and the Resonator—each a step from dependency to contribution. Over tea with a neighbour, I mused— "It's not one thing, but all together"—and she nodded. My chest, once a battleground, now breathes free; my mind, once shadowed, shines clear—a journey from 5 pounds 7 ounces to this, nearly eight decades on.

This complete design is no mere personal triumph—it is a blueprint for dignity. At 81, I stand as evidence—hospitals see me no more, my kin bear no weight, and I aid others: over a thousand minds, over 200 bodies. You need not falter as I did at 52—draining those around you—but may forge this circle instead. Clear your mind with RONE, quell your foes with the Resonator, eat wisely, move daily, tend your needs—forty is your moment, before or after, to choose renewal over ruin. It took me decades—born frail, faltering midlife—to discern this path, yet it sustains me now, a testament to what you too might claim. Live well, spare others your strain, extend a hand—it is yours, should you choose to grasp it.

Chapter 7

Still Going Strong and Healthy

Here I sit at 81, in my armchair with a cup of tea— green tea, marvelling that I remain to recount this tale—a journey from a frail beginning to a vigour I scarcely imagined possible. Born in 1943, at 5 pounds and 7 ounces, I emerged jaundiced, skin peeling, my mother's wartime anxieties from nursing her sister's wounds from a bomb during the last three months of her pregnancy, imprinting a tension science later affirmed: distress in the womb marks a child enduringly. By eighteen months, asthma had seized me—breaths wheezing, chest tight—my mother keeping vigil, unaware her unrest echoed within me, my father reaching into my cot to confirm my survival, crafting cardboard splints to curb my scratching of eczematous skin.

In 1948, our National Health Service doctor suggested to my parents, they send me to Ventnor's convalescent home—five years among fellow asthmatics, our days hushed, my stammer silencing me further. At eleven, the eleven-plus exam yielded a middling result—an oral test followed, where three examiners spoke my name and answers as I nodded or shook my head, passing me in a curious charade. Grammar school saw summers lost to coughing, departing at sixteen with one O-level in English Language, pneumonia thwarting the rest.

At eighteen, I joined DER as their youngest outside engineer driving house to house, repairing television sets —a task I savoured until restlessness led me away after two years. Adulthood unravelled chaotically—three marriages, the first two barren from my own lack, my first wife's and my own insecurity met with shouting matches I failed to fathom, the second lost to my poor conduct, until a vitamin at fifty sparked life with my third, yielding two children now in their thirties. Yet my temper sundered that too by 1993, leaving me a man adrift, my distant offspring my sole tether. Driving instruction over thirty years offered solace—women cautious, men bold, until the birth pill in the 1960s turned ladies daring, a shift I linked to, proven decades later—a quiet vindication. By 52, in 1995, I was a ruin—lungs at half capacity, teeth gone, hips arthritic, pneumonia twice, chest infections biannual, mild COPD from a 1959 doctor's folly to smoke. Alone, I weighed ending it—my children's memory restrained me—yet I burdened all: doctors, kin, society.

Then came renewal—late 1990s, past 50, a chance encounter at a jive dance session, where I watched rather than danced, led a kind lady to invite me to a therapy workshop. There, Emotional Freedom Technique—EFT—entered my life, a method of tapping body points to ease distress. Seated in my armchair with its manual, I dulled my hip pain, a flicker of hope in my gloom. That spark ignited a quest—two years of inquiry, scouring a nascent internet and ancient texts from China and Egypt, seeking a vital energy within us. Modern medicine dismissed it, but I pressed on, aiding friends and pupils with EFT—sometimes it lifted burdens, sometimes not—until 2000, when I crafted RONE Therapy—Removal of Negative Emotions—a method born of patience, designed to banish distress with certainty, one session sufficed: I would sit with an individual—over a thousand since—asking not for their full tale, but the emotion—anger, fear, guilt—weighing their heart. Clear instructions, spoken once, guided them to focus on the feeling of each emotion, then they dissolved—Mr. Thompson's for his son—leaving clarity where shadows reigned. RONE's precision astonished me—my hip pain, bone on bone, vanished for twelve years, a thousand others followed: Mr. Carter's lingering ache from a neighbour's slight, Miss Evans' chest tightened by lost love, countless men vexed by temper, women worn by worry, elderly folk bowed by regret—all lifted, save two who clung to pain for gain or excuse. I learned to speak first, ensuring their will to heal—Mr. Thompson's tears, after eight years of back pain from a ladder fall, affirmed it: guilt for rejecting his wayward son, not doctors' failures, held his torment. Over tea, he stood, pain gone, a truth I've seen often repeated: pain past a year is emotion's echo—anger at myself, once my shield, now my lesson. half a minute to sustain—RONE freed my mind at 57, a cornerstone of this renewal, its reach a testament to simplicity's power.

Yet my body lingered—lungs rasping—until 2018, at 74, a Ukrainian lady's bio-resonance dud spurred Clark's The Cure, a shed Zapper becoming my Resonator— quelling infections, restoring smell, over 200 lives like my friend at 90 spared.
Why had I faltered, and how did I rise? I found the way, but you may not. Consider

this, trillions of bacteria from birth via mother lie dormant—Why not consume us at once? It's pH—1 to 14, 7 neutral, 7.3 healthy—oxygen-rich, keeping them asleep. Over 40, they wake—aches, then organs, then death. What drops pH? Not just food—stress, my 25 years of RONE affirm. Cortisol from worry sours blood, cells, waking bacteria—my shouting, my temper, my 52 ruin.

Forty's the hinge—before, youth holds pH; after, neglect stirs them. A century ago, 40 was life's span—sportsmen fade then, dementia's bacterial scent begins, as mine did, reversed by the Resonator. Three ladies under 40 at a fair—cancer, pH below 5.5—yet no aches; over 40, my clients bore both, until RONE and Resonator intervened. At 81, my IHeart reads arteries at 54, heart 58 beats a minute—proof of reversal: RONE cleared stress, Resonator quelled bacteria, diet shed two stone in three weeks (How I Lost 2 Stone in 3 Weeks), walks and vitamins bolstered, blood type tuned—O fiery, A stubborn—my circle complete.

This isn't my triumph alone—over 200 Resonators, a thousand RONE sessions—doctors see me no more, kin bear no load. Big firms scorn it—no pill profits; authorities demand proof, ignoring decades of lives like Mr. Carter's laugh, Miss Evans' toast, Mr. Thompson's tears—yet I challenge any to disprove it. After reading some may think the Resonator is all they need, but there are many who have used the Resonator for pain, only to find that it was emotional.

40 is your choice—before, mind falters, but the body holds; after 40, stress wakes the reaper's little helpers unless you act. RONE, lifts your spirit in hours, a skill yours to keep; Resonator, kills bacteria, parasites, viruses—no drugs needed. What if there were none there to consume us? How long would we live healthily? Eat wisely, move, tend yourself, a few vitamins—my 52 burden,

became 81 strength. You need not drain others—rise, help your fellows, keep the reaper waiting, destroy his little helpers. At 81, I'm proof—frail to firm, a path yours if you take it.

A wealthy philanthropist could herald RONE and the Resonator —your legacy outshining all.

"Good health is not everything, but without it, everything is nothing" — Socrates

ISBN 9780956793836

Notes

www.ingramcontent.com/pod-product-compliance
Ingram Content Group UK Ltd.
Pitfield, Milton Keynes, MK11 3LW, UK
UKHW041854040425
5323UKWH00026B/92

9 780956 793836